THE MODEL BODY PLAN

A Motivational Weight Loss & Fitness
Plan That Strips Away the Fat

AESHA WAKS

Order this book online at www.trafford.com
or email orders@trafford.com

Most Trafford titles are also available at major online book retailers.

EDITED BY: Chris Northrop

COVER PHOTO BY: Lenka Drstakova

Print information available on the last page.

ISBN: 978-1-4907-6879-3 (sc)
ISBN: 978-1-4907-6881-6 (hc)
ISBN: 978-1-4907-6880-9 (e)

Library of Congress Control Number: 2016900299

Trafford rev. 02/04/2016

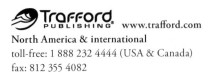 www.trafford.com

North America & international
toll-free: 1 888 232 4444 (USA & Canada)
fax: 812 355 4082

CONTENTS

PART I
DIET

PART II
EXERCISE & FITNESS

PART III
LIFESTYLE

PART IV
INSPIRATION

PART V
4-WEEK JOURNAL

- DIET
- EXERCISE & FITNESS
- LIFESTYLE
- INSPIRATIONAL

DEDICATION

I dedicate this book to my late mother Mindy Waks, my late grandmother Sylvia Metzger and my family in heaven. Their unconditional love gave me the courage to be myself and explore my dreams.

ACKNOWLEDGEMENTS

Thank you Chris Northrop for helping me put my thoughts onto paper. Chris, you have been the source of my greatest inspiration to achieve the impossible. I would also like to thank my family and friends for their ongoing encouragement and support, you all know who you are.

Some special thanks:

Miri Ben-Ari
Thea Conners
Renoly Santiago
Lenka Drastokova
Antoine Verglas
Edward Jahn
Marilyn Krochmal Gelfand
Collin Slattery
Sergio Murillo
Brian Greene
Robert Pjetri
Jonas Borra
Andre Joseph
Choco Llama
Donna Murphy
Jessie May
Israel Waks
Geffen Waks
The Mulvanertys
Steven Leff
Laurie Meadoff
Conrad Szumilas
Andy Estonia

PREFACE

From the time I was a teenager, throughout my early 20's, I struggled with a slew of eating disorders. I battled borderline anorexia, nighttime binging and was obsessed with working out. Guilt led to stress, which led to other problems such as acid reflux.

At my lowest, I weighted only 90 lbs. My mother was extremely concerned with my health. She threatened to check me into a hospital. I promised her that if she gave me some time I would figure it out on my own. I was fortunate to have an understanding and loving mother who believed in me.

My initial goal was to gain 10 lbs., however, I feared that if I began to put on weight I wouldn't be able to control it. This fear led to strange eating patterns. I'd eat a box of cookies in the middle of the night, feel guilty and then fast the next day. I thought that by eating junk food I'd gain weight, but that wasn't the case. It didn't seem to matter what I ate or when I ate it, but rather the amount of calories I was eating each day. The box of cookies had fewer than 1,000 calories, so I wasn't gaining any weight. My mother wasn't seeing any changes, so I had to force myself to eat more. As I initially feared, I gained more than 10 lbs. I needed to become educated on how to control my weight, so I set out to learn everything there was to know about weight management, health and fitness. I began to read a lot on the subject and started working with a personal trainer.

My personal trainer provided me with an effective workout routine as well as a popular diet plan. I really liked what I was learning in the gym, however, I found the diet to be too strict and regimented for my liking. If I strayed from the rules of the plan, my trainer would accuse me of "cheating!" I didn't like feeling like a cheater. I wanted some leeway. I wanted choices and didn't want to have to give up the foods I loved. I was determined to find a way to create a plan that worked for me.

I researched and read popular weight loss books and fitness magazines. I feverishly took notes in my journal, cross referenced materials, highlighted key points and even sketched out graphs. I started to notice patterns and began to distinguish scientific facts from fads. At this point I felt that I had gained enough knowledge and experience to compile an effective diet and exercise plan.

The first version of my plan was written as an essay. I submitted it to my professor while I was working toward completing my Bachelor of Science degree at New York University (NYU). She loved it and encouraged me to continue to develop my plan and eventually turn it into a book.

This plan has worked for me, and my clients. I'm proud to share it with you.

INTRODUCTION

Before you begin *The Model Body Plan*, you're going to need to go out and buy a couple of things:

- Scale *(to log your current weight and track future weight loss)*
- Tape Measure *(to log your current and future measurements)*

I also recommend the following tools to help you measure food and properly track your daily caloric intake:

- Food Scale
- Measuring Cups
- Measuring Spoons
- Calorie Counter Reference Guide

It's important to log your current weight and measurements as well as two desired goal weights. The first is a realistic goal weight and the second is an ultimate ideal weight, which can be used to motivate you. I advise setting a realistic goal, because if one looses too much weight too quickly an array of health problems could arise. It's quite possible that you can achieve your realistic goal by simply making a few minor changes to your lifestyle and habits. Reaching your ultimate ideal goal weight will take greater will power and commitment as well as a better understanding of the dieting process.

As you work toward your goals, be happy with yourself and know that you are in control of what you will look like from this point on. You're only as thin as the effort you are willing to put into it. It all boils down to choices and the choice is yours!

To help get started, I've provided you with a Weight & Measurement Log. Write down your current weight and measurements, realistic goal weight and ultimate ideal goal weight.

I've also provided you with a 3-Day Starter Journal. It's important to jot down your current eating and drinking patterns. Over the course of the next three days you will need to log the times you eat and/or drink, what you eat and/or drink, how many calories you consume when you eat and/or drink and how many times a day you eat and/or drink.

After you've logged your 3-day diet, add up your total calories from each day and divide that number by three. This is roughly your current daily caloric intake. Now take that number and minus 250 calories. If you desire faster weight loss results, you can minus 500 calories from your current daily caloric intake. Whichever option you choose will be your new goal number of calories to hit each day, if your doctor is fine with that.

Good luck!

WEIGHT & MEASUREMENT LOG

Date _____

WEIGHTS

Current Weight _____

Realistic Goal Weight _____

Ultimate Ideal Goal Weight _____

MEASUREMENTS

Height _____

Chest _____

Waist _____

Hips _____

3-DAY STARTER JOURNAL

DAY 1

MEAL #	TIME	FOOD / DRINK	CALORIES

Day 1 – Total Calories = _____

DAY 2

MEAL #	TIME	FOOD / DRINK	CALORIES

Day 2 – Total Calories = _____

DAY 3

MEAL #	TIME	FOOD / DRINK	CALORIES

Day 3 – Total Calories = _____

Now that you've completed your 3-Day Starter Journal, add up the total calories from all three days and divide that number by three. This is your approximate daily caloric intake. Log this number below:

Daily Caloric Intake Number = _____

If you'd like to begin on a comfortable track to loosing weight, minus 250 calories from your daily caloric intake number. If you'd rather opt to begin on a faster path to reaching your goal, then subtract 500 calories from your daily caloric intake number, if you and your health care physician are fine with that. Log that number below:

New Daily Caloric Intake Goal Number = _____

PART I

DIET

Chapter 1

COMPARATIVE PLANS

Throughout the years, I've researched and read many diet books and tried most of the popular plans. While there is merit to these plans, they have failed me. I've found these plans to be too rigid. If you break one rule, the entire house of cards collapses. I was left feeling guilty and it brought me back to square one. Here's an overview of some of the more popular diet philosophies that I've researched and tried in the past:

Traditional Plan

This is the most common plan. Simply put, you eat three meals—breakfast, lunch and dinner—and three snacks a day. For women, combined calories from meals and snacks should not exceed approximately 1,200 calories. Men can add a few hundred calories more to this number. Height and weight does factor into the exact daily caloric count. While this is a great starting point (and I understand the value of eating three meals a day), I am not a morning person and thus rarely eat breakfast. I also felt it was a bit rigid to commit to eating three snacks everyday of the week.

Points System

With this mainstream popular approach foods are assigned point values. It's like going to the casino and trading in money for clay chips, but more complicated. At a casino, if I have 100 dollars to gamble with then I have a few options. I could trade in my money for twenty $5 red chips or four $25 green chips or one $100 black chip. It's pretty clear-cut. However, with this point plan the options are so much greater, because there are thousands of different combinations of foods and meals available to choose from. In order to grasp the system and accurately count the points it is encouraged to use a points manual and buy foods sold by the company that created this plan.

When I go out for a slice of pizza different pizzerias use different flours, different amounts of cheese, etc., thus the calories could differ. It was extremely hard to transfer these foods into points unless I was buying this company's pre-fixed meals. I didn't want to be limited to their way.

Food Combination

The philosophy behind this plan is to combine proteins, carbohydrates and fats to create balanced meals or snacks that you eat every 2–6 hours, 4–5 times a day. While I found this diet easier to comprehend than a point system, it had flaws. I live in a big city. I am on the go and often eat out. I found it very hard to eat balanced meals and/or snacks 4-5 times everyday. Sometimes I only had time for two meals a day and though it's not ideal I still lost weight. Another issue I had was that I was told I was "cheating" if I wanted to grab a bag of fries or a yogurt on the go. I became frustrated and started feeling guilty because I was breaking the rules.

Dividing Food Groups

The structure of this diet is to divide food groups. Optimally, eat fruits in the morning, carbohydrates throughout the day and proteins in the evening. The idea behind this diet is that this type of eating pattern will get your body use to digesting certain foods at certain times, which can promote weight loss. Each food group takes different amounts of time to digest. For instance, fruits take less time to digest than proteins and that's why it's suggested to eat only fruits in the morning. You are not limited to the amount of calories you can consume on a daily basis, however, eating less will lead to greater weight loss. If you divide food groups it can work, however, the rigidness wasn't for me. If I wanted to have a hot dog for example, that wouldn't fit in anywhere because a hot dog combines protein (meat) and carbohydrates (bun). This plan doesn't leave enough room for flexibility. As soon as I bent the rules, I gained the weight right back.

Vegetarian / Vegan /Pescetarian

The vegetarian diet consists of primarily vegetables. While vegetarians don't eat meat, some may eat animal byproducts such as milk, eggs and cheese. The vegan diet is a stricter version of a vegetarian diet. Vegans do not eat meat or animal byproducts. The pescetarian diet consists of eating primarily fish and other seafood. Pescetarians do not eat the meat of other animals, but incorporate vegetables, nuts and animal byproducts such as honey into their diet.

The practice of these diets is both humane and healthy for the body. I tried these diets, but couldn't keep it up for the long haul. When I began incorporating meat into my diet, my body struggled to digest the protein. I gained all the weight right back. I commend anyone who chooses one of these diets. Personally, I was not able to fully commit to this lifestyle, but I do incorporate organic and free-range meals into my diet as often as possible.

All Protein

The all protein diet became a mainstream fad years ago. Simply put, it encourages the consumption of proteins and fats. Vegetables are allowed in limited consumption, but carbohydrates are discouraged, especially at the start of the diet. Eventually, you can begin to incorporate carbohydrates in very limited amounts. While this diet works, it's unrealistic for most people to eat little to no carbohydrates. I couldn't imagine not being able to enjoy a bowl of pasta, a bagel or a donut. I knew I would not be able to keep this rigid all protein diet up. As expected, as soon as I craved a carbohydrate the weight came right back and I felt like a failure.

Conclusion

By researching and trying all of these diets I learned a lot. While there are many positive aspects to these plans, I found all lacked the flexibility I needed to feel good about the process of loosing and maintaining my weight. I became set on creating my own plan. I took into account commonalities and differences of popular diets as well as proven scientific facts versus fads. I developed a structure to my diet that leaves room for flexibility so you can feel good about yourself while you're loosing weight. I am confident that my plan will help you reach your model body.

Chapter 2

AN INTRODUCTION TO DIETING

By now you've completed your 3-Day Starter Journal and logged the results. You've determined your daily caloric intake then subtracted either 250 calories or 500 calories (if you are opting to attempt a faster path to reaching your goal). This number is your new daily caloric intake goal to meet each day. Ultimately, you must work toward shrinking the size of your stomach, thus I can't stress enough how important it is to meet your new daily caloric intake goal.

Make a decision whether you are dieting simply to lose weight or to lose weight and live a healthier lifestyle. It is possible to lose weight while still eating junk food as long as you don't exceed your daily caloric intake goal. If you crave sweets or are a fast food junkie, then it might be beneficial to learn to love healthier foods, because vegetables are a staple of *The Model Body Plan*.

Get into the routine of eating a few small meals a day. Four meals a day is optimal, but if your schedule doesn't permit it or if special occasions arise then 3-5 meals is okay. Keep in mind, the more meals you eat in a day the smaller the portions must be to avoid exceeding your daily caloric intake goal.

Ideally your meals should consist of vegetables, proteins, carbohydrates, and fats. The reason for this is to balance your blood sugar and keep you full.

When eating your meals do your best to eat slowly. Typically people who eat fast consume more food in a shorter amount of time, because it takes the brain approximately 20 minutes to register that the stomach is full. There is less of a chance you will go back for seconds if you slow down when eating a meal.

Try your best to space meals apart by at least two hours. This will give your stomach time to digest the food and burn some of the calories off in the process.

Dieting Overview

Here is a short list of key points that make up the structure of *The Model Body Plan:*

- Subtract 250-500 calories from your daily caloric intake
- 4 meals a day (ideally)
- If you are stuck on using titles, you can opt. to use breakfast/ lunch/dinner/snack instead of meal (1/2/3/4) for example
- Balanced meals consisting of proteins, carbohydrates and fats (ideally)
- Wait at least 2 hours between meals
- 50 calories or less is a freebie
- Unlimited Water and Vegetables

In the following chapters we will discuss my plan in more detail, but first let's clear up some dieting myths.

Dieting Myths

Don't feel guilty or fall victim to dieting myths or old wives tales. Guilt can lead to stress and stress can lead to overeating. When I work with a new client I make it a point to clear up some of these myths. Here are some examples of dieting myths:

Client: I can't eat certain foods, because it will make me fat.
Me: *Untrue. You can eat whatever you'd like as long as don't exceed your daily caloric intake goal.*

Client: As long as I eat healthy I will lose weight.
Me: *Untrue. While eating healthy is a bonus to losing weight, it is not the deciding factor whether or not you will shed pounds. Fish, fruits, granola bars and whole wheat bread are all examples of healthy foods that when eaten in excess will lead to weight gain. Healthy foods have calories too. The key to losing weight is eating in moderation and meeting your daily caloric intake goal.*

Client: I can't eat late at night or I will gain weight.
Me: *Untrue. As long as you have not exceeded your daily caloric intake goal you can eat anytime of the day you'd like.*

Client: If I eat fruits all the time I will lose weight.
Me: *Untrue. Unlike vegetables, fruits have calories and many are high in sugars. Fruits are beneficial and can help you lose weight when eaten as a replacement to a carbohydrate (or eaten on it's own as part of your daily caloric intake), but eating fruits all the time will not necessarily help you lose weight.*

Client: As long as a beverage has zero fat I can drink as much as I want and won't gain weight.
Me: *Untrue. Just because a beverage, such as some brands of ice tea, has zero fat doesn't mean it has zero calories. Fat and calories are two separate entities. You can still gain weight from consuming fat free beverages that contain calories.*

I've heard all sorts of dieting myths and most are simply untrue. Do not let myths worry you. Focus your efforts on meeting your daily caloric intake goal. A great way to do this is to eat lots of vegetables.

Chapter 3

VEGETABLES

Vegetables are a staple of *The Model Body Plan*. Vegetables do not contain countable calories, thus you can eat as many as you'd like as often as you'd like. Roughage helps to push other foods and toxins through your body, which helps eliminate fat and waste. Eating hearty portions of vegetable will help you lose weight, because your stomach will remain full leaving little room for fatty foods that could push you past your daily caloric intake goal.

Here are some useful tips for incorporating more vegetables into your diet:

- Green, leafy vegetables are optimum for losing weight.
- Bulk up your meals with vegetables. Instead of eating a bowl of pasta with bread or a plate of chicken and rice, cut the portion of carbohydrates and proteins in half and add spinach, broccoli or a salad. This shrinks the number of calories, creates a more balanced meal and will fill up your stomach.
- Keep a pot of steamed vegetables handy. Graze on it throughout the day.
- Stock up on raw vegetables. Carry carrots and celery sticks with you at all times.
- Grab a celery juice. It's a great energizer and a healthy alternative to sodas that are loaded with sugars and calories.
- Substitute fattening deserts such as cookies and cakes with sweet vegetable freebies (i.e.: sweet summer squash with

cinnamon). Your sweet tooth will be satisfied and your stomach will thank you.

Vegetable Fasts

I understand that for some of you vegetables are not the most exciting part of a meal, however, vegetables are a vital component to losing weight. A great way to get your mind and body use to vegetables is to jump right in with a vegetable and vegetable juice fast. It will cleanse your body of toxins, energize you and fill your stomach with foods free of countable calories. Try it out for a day or so, then begin to incorporate other foods into your diet over the next few days. I've always found this approach to be most effective. It's like jumping into a cold swimming pool rather than trying to walk in step by step. The initial shock is hard, but after only a few moments your body acclimates. Before you know it, you will have built the foundation of a stable diet. Consult with your doctor if you opt to begin *The Model Body Plan* with a vegetable and vegetable juice fast, or any fast at any point for that matter.

Chapter 4

FREEBIES

A freebie is any food, beverage or condiment that is 50 calories or less. Like vegetables, it is a staple component of *The Model Body Plan*. Eating half an apple or sipping on a small box of juice is a great way to revive your metabolism throughout the day. Another reason why I encourage freebies is because your body will naturally burn off 50 calories in a short amount of time, thus it does not count toward your daily caloric intake goal. A freebie is also a great way to satisfy a craving for a particular food or drink. For example, coffee with cream counts as a freebie. If you have a sweet tooth, then you can grab a lollypop or enjoy a bite of chocolate cake. Prefer salty foods? Grab a pickle. It's a freebie!

Chapter 5

VITAMINS & SUPPLEMENTS

Most people do not get the proper amount of nutrients required to sustain a healthy body and lifestyle. I recommend incorporating multivitamins and/or herbal supplements into your daily diet. I personally prefer chewable multivitamins. According to the Supplement Facts listed on the label of a bottle of Centrum MultiGummies, the recommended daily dosage is two gummies. Two gummies contains only 10 calories making it a freebie. Multivitamins serve as a great supplement that will energize you throughout the day. Vitamins and supplements will also boost your immune system and help fight the common cold.

Chapter 6

HONEY & APPLE CIDER VINEGAR

Honey is a natural sweetener that is low in calories and promotes good health. A teaspoon of honey contains approximately 20 calories making it an ideal freebie (when eaten on it's own). Spread it on toast, add a teaspoon or two to a cup of hot tea or drizzle it on granola. It will satisfy your sweet tooth and help fight the common cold.

In addition to honey, I suggest keeping a bottle of apple cider vinegar in your home. Most brands are low to no calories. Apple cider vinegar can be used as an ingredient in salad dressing. Add a small splash of unfiltered apple cider vinegar to a glass of water to help boost immune function. Health benefits could include everything from helping to eliminate nail fungus to fighting the flu.

Chapter 7

WATER

I can't stress enough how important it is to consume generous amounts of water each day. Water will keep you hydrated and push toxins through your body. Like most vegetables and freebies, water does not count toward your daily caloric intake so you can have as much as you'd like as often as you'd like.

Chop fruit such as cantaloupe or vegetables such as cucumbers and add it to a pitcher of ice water. This makes a fragrant and fresh summer drink. As long as you don't eat the fruit, it's also free of countable calories.

Seltzer water contains zero calories and is a great alternative for those of you who prefer carbonated beverages. Add a splash of fruit juice to create a tasty low calorie drink that counts as a freebie.

For those of you on the go, powdered drink mixes, such as Crystal Light, are convenient and have little to no countable calories. Whatever option you choose, be sure to stay hydrated throughout the day.

Some research recommends that one should drink at least eight, 8-ounce glasses of water a day. I encourage you to make water a key component of your diet.

Chapter 8

JUNK FOOD

While junk food typically contains more fat content than fat free foods, junk food will not necessarily increase your weight (when eaten in moderation). On *The Model Body Plan* we focus on counting calories, not fat, and both junk food and healthy food contain calories. It's your choice whether you want to lose weight and become healthier or simply shed pounds.

In Chapter 2, under the Dieting Myths section I touched upon this topic. Here's an example to add additional clarity to the subject. A burger, fries and soda from a fast food chain has a comparable amount of calories to a grilled chicken sandwich, baked potato and juice prepared at home. While the latter is a healthier option, both contain roughly the same amount of calories. As long as you hit your daily caloric intake goal, you will not gain weight from eating the junk food option.

While eating junk food might not necessarily increase your weight, it could leave you feeling lethargic and unmotivated. Unhealthy fats found in junk food, such as lard, could lead to high cholesterol. You might also get hungrier faster after consuming junk food, making it harder for you to meet your daily caloric intake goal.

Ask yourself, do I want to lose weight and live a healthier lifestyle or simply weigh less? The choice is yours!

Chapter 9

MEAL REPLACEMENTS

Based on a standard 1200 calorie diet, broken up into 4 equal 300 calorie meals. An ideal meal consists of 2 carbohydrates to 1 protein to 1 fat (that is approximately ¼ the amount of calories as the protein). An ideal meal that totals approximately 300 calories could consist of 1 cup of brown rice (carbohydrate) that contains approximately 180 calories and 2 oz. of tuna (protein) that contains approximately 90 calories and 1 teaspoon of olive oil (fat) that contains approximately 25 calories. So for every 200 calories of carbohydrates you should eat approximately 100 calories of protein and 25 calories of fat.

Now that you have an understanding of an ideal meal, let's define the term meal replacement. A meal replacement is the action of substituting one or more components (carbohydrate, protein, fat) of an ideal meal with a different one, while keeping the total calories of that meal the same. By keeping the total calories of the meal the same.

Replacing components of meals is another way in which my plan differs from other popular diets that I mentioned in Chapter 1. I am offering you the flexibility to make your own choices as long as you can still meet your daily caloric intake goal. You don't have to completely cut out the foods you love, but keep in mind that if you eat a piece of cake you might have to skip a meal, eat two half meals or bulk up on vegetables the rest of the day to avoid consuming too many calories.

Meal replacements have worked for me as well as for many of my clients. You should not feel guilty if you want to treat yourself to the food you love. You know yourself better than anyone. If you have an addictive personality and feel that by reaching for a sweet treat it might put you over the edge, then consider cutting these types of foods out completely. I'm leaving it up to you!

Chapter 10

DIET EXAMPLES

Through years of research and experience, I've found that with most diets the recommended daily caloric intake goal is approximately 1,200 calories for women and 1,500 calories for men. Other factors such as your height and weight (at the start of your diet) as well as your previous eating habits will ultimately determine your exact daily caloric intake goal.

Below I've listed two diet examples. The first is what a day could look like for a person whose daily caloric intake goal totals 1,200 calories. The second example is a diet with a daily caloric intake cap of 1,500 calories. Meal 1 is an example of an ideal meal. Meal 2 is an example of a meal replacement. Meal 3 is an example of a healthy smaller meal. Meal 4 is an example of a junk food meal. Keep in mind you can add vegetables (preferably green vegetables) to any meal, because vegetables consist of little to no countable calories. You may also incorporate water, seltzer water and freebies into your diet throughout the day. Remember, freebies are any food, beverage or condiment that totals 50 calories or less.

Diet Example 1

Meal 1 – Ideal Meal
1 cup of oatmeal – 150 calories
1 cup of skim milk – 90 calories

1 teaspoon of butter – 30 calories
½ glass of orange juice – 50 calories
= 320 calories

Meal 2 – Meal Replacement
1 cup of brown rice – 215 calories
1 teaspoon of olive oil – 25 calories
1 teaspoon of soy sauce - freebie
Unlimited green vegetable - freebie
1 cup of green tea – freebie
= 240 calories

Meal 3 – Healthy Smaller Meal
1 apple – 95 calories
1 slice of American cheese – 105 calories
1 bottle of seltzer water – freebie
= 200 calories

Meal 4 – Junk Food Meal
1 slice of pizza – 285 calories
1 can of ginger ale – 125 calories
= 410 calories

Daily Caloric Intake Total = 1,170 calories

Diet Example 2

Meal 1 – Ideal Meal
2 eggs - 140 calories
1 teaspoon of butter - 30 calories
2 slices of whole wheat bread - 140 calories
1 coffee - freebie
= 310 calories

Meal 2 – Meal Replacement
1 3 oz. can of tuna – 150 calories
2 teaspoons of mayo – 60 calories

3 leaves of lettuce – freebie
1 bottle of water – freebie
1 oz. of cashew nuts – 150 calories
= 360 calories

Meal 3 – Healthy Smaller Meal
1 yogurt – 90 calories
1 small box of apple juice – 60 calories
= 150 calories

Meal 4 – Junk Food Meal
1 cheeseburger – 300 calories
1 bag of small fries – 230 calories
1 small fountain soda – 140 calories
= 670 calories

Daily Caloric Intake Total = 1,490 calories

The calories in the above diet examples are estimates. Calories in foods and beverages differ from brand to brand. As you start your diet, be sure to reference the nutrient facts located on the packages of most foods. Nutrition information is also available at most restaurants and can be researched on the Internet as well.

Chapter 11

AVOIDING HEALTH PROBLEMS WHEN DIETING

When improperly dieting, health and other problems could arise. Here are a few examples to be aware of:

Depression

Depression can lead to overeating. Overeating can lead to exceeding your daily caloric intake goal, which could then lead to feelings of failure. Stay in high spirits and trust that you can meet your goals. Dieting is challenging, however, on *The Model Body Plan* I am giving you the flexibility to eat what you want when you want, as long as you meet your daily caloric intake goal. Don't be hard on yourself. Losing weight takes time, but you can do it. Reward yourself once a week with that piece of chocolate cake you crave (you just may need to replace at least two meals for it).

Dry Skin

Daily routines, such as moisturizing your skin, could greatly help during the dieting process. Make sure to hydrate your skin by drinking plenty of water.

Acid Reflux

While acid reflux can be caused by certain foods, I developed it from stress. I felt ashamed that I could not maintain rigid diets that I tried in the past. This was my greatest motivation to crafting a stress-free diet plan.

When one is active and happy, serotonin is created, which relaxes the body and aids in digestion. Do your best to not stress yourself during the dieting process. Remain calm and committed. Be proud of even the smallest accomplishments. Losing as little as one pound a week is a great success. Smile and stay positive!

Gallstones

Gallstones can be a side effect of losing too much weight too quickly. While most diets recommend a daily caloric intake goal of 1,200 calories for women and 1,500 calories for men this is unrealistic if your daily caloric intake prior to dieting is a significantly higher number. As I mentioned at the start of this book, consult with your doctor and simply subtract 250-500 calories from your daily caloric intake prior to dieting and that is your new goal number to hit each day. If after several months you are meeting and maintaining your goal, then you may consider subtracting additional calories from your daily caloric intake. I can't stress enough how losing too much weight too quickly could lead to health problems. If a problem arises, be sure to consult your primary care physician. Your health means more than the speed at which you lose weight.

Chapter 12

RESOURCES TO FINDING NUTRITIONAL INFORMATION

Apps

Restaurants as well as popular fast food chains offer apps that contain nutritional facts. These apps can be downloaded (often for free) to your smartphone or tablet device. The McDonald's app includes detailed nutritional information including calories, ingredients and allergens. If you are looking for a healthier fast food alternative, Chipotle is a great option. Chipotle's app is fully customizable. You can build your own meal, select your own ingredients then determine your total calories. For coffee lovers, the Starbucks app offers detailed nutritional information that lists the milligrams of caffeine found in their beverages. Modern technology has made it easier than ever to count your calories.

Websites

Many restaurants offer detailed nutritional information on their websites. Applebee's offers an easily readable nutrition chart that you can download to your computer. I encourage you to search your favorite restaurants on the Internet. It is free, convenient and a great reference tool.

Reference Guides

If you are an old soul like me and still read books, reference guides that list the caloric content of thousands of foods are available at major book retailers such as Barnes & Noble. These guides are a great resource when dieting.

Packaging

For those of you who enjoy cooking at home, most foods found at your local grocery store list calories, serving sizes and other nutritional information on the packages.

We live in a world with an abundance of information at our fingertips. Apps, websites, reference guides and information found on packaging are great resources to get you started. Once you get into the habit of becoming familiar with nutritional information, the process will become second nature to you. You'll be on your way to achieving your goals.

PART II

EXERCISE & FITNESS

Chapter 13

AN INTRODUCTION TO EXERCISE & FITNESS

Meeting your daily caloric intake goal and following *The Model Body Plan's* diet structure will help you meet your weight loss goals. I also strongly encourage you to incorporate an exercise and fitness routine into your weekly schedule. This will aid in the weight loss process, boost your overall energy, build muscle mass and keep you lean and tone.

Earlier in this book I explained and gave examples of an ideal meal. To refresh, an ideal meal consists of 2 carbohydrates to 1 protein to 1 fat (that is approximately ¼ the amount of calories as the protein). I've also given examples of other meal options such as meal replacements, junk food meals and healthy smaller meals. You could lose weight with any of these options as long as you meet your daily caloric intake goal, however, your body mass index (BMI) or body fat percentage (BFP) might be different based on your dietary choices.

What does this mean? Without getting too scientific it basically means that two people can be the same height and weight, but look different based on dietary and exercise choices. A person who eats primarily ideal meals and incorporates exercise and fitness into their weekly routines could appear more muscularly defined and/or tone than a person who eats primarily junk food meals and does not exercise. Both persons can consume the same amount of calories each day, but the second person's body will hold more body fat (because of dietary choices and lack of exercise), thus could appear soft and less defined.

At the beginning of this book, I advised that before you start my plan you should decide whether you are dieting to simply shed pounds or to lose weight and be healthier. I will pose a similar choice now. Is your goal to simply shed pounds or to lose weight and achieve a desirable, fit appearance? If it is the latter option, you will find the following chapters useful.

Weightlifting, cardio and calisthenics are important components to achieving your desired look. Exercise and fitness builds muscle mass and keeps you lean and tone. Incorporating ideal meals and healthier food options will increase energy levels, build strength and boost your endurance to ensure you get the most out of your workout sessions.

Chapter 14

WEIGHTLIFTING

Weightlifting builds and strengthens muscles, releases endorphins, boosts energy levels and will make you feel better about yourself overall. Before you begin a weightlifting routine, ask yourself the following questions:

- Which exercises would I like to incorporate into my routine?
- How many sets (number of cycles) will I complete for each exercise?
- How many reps (number of times I lift and lower the weight) will I complete in a set?

There are several weightlifting exercises that vary in difficulty to choose from as you craft your custom workout routine. I recommend selecting 3 to 4 exercises for each large body part and 2 to 3 exercises for each small body part. If you choose the smaller number, be sure to do an extra set of reps. Large and small body parts will be discussed in greater detail later in this chapter.

Once you've determined which exercises you'd like to incorporate into your routine, next decide how many sets you'd like to complete for each exercise. I personally recommend 3 to 4 sets per exercise for large body parts and 2 to 3 sets per exercise for small body parts. Once you've completed a set, it's best to rest. If you are in a time crunch, complete a set then switch to the other body part you are working on that day and keep rotating between body parts.

Now determine how many reps you will complete in each set. I recommend targeting 10 reps per set. If you can only complete 8 reps in a set that's fine, don't beat yourself up, but I encourage you to set your goal number at 10.

The general rule of thumb is that if you lift heavier weights less times you will build mass, whereas if you lift lighter weights many times your body will become more defined and tone. Unless you are an Olympic dead lifter, I do not promote lifting extreme amounts of weight a couple of times nor do I feel it's beneficial to complete a ridiculous amount of sets lifting a very light weight. I believe in balance. Do the best you can do without hurting yourself.

I crafted a weightlifting routine that focuses on working muscles in different body parts on different days throughout week. The body is broken down into two major sections consisting of large and small parts.

<u>Large Parts</u>
- Chest
- Back
- Legs

<u>Small Parts</u>
- Biceps
- Triceps
- Shoulders

It is optimal to workout 3 days a week. On each day pick 2 body parts to workout. It could be 1 large body part and 1 small body part or 2 large body parts, etc. Mix it up from week to week to break up the monotony or keep it the same to maintain a structured routine. Whatever combination works best for you is fine as long as you work each of the 6 parts once a week.

Most of my workouts last between an hour and an hour and half and consist not only of weightlifting, but also cardio and calisthenics, which we will discuss in the following chapters. Typically I incorporate 3 to 4 different exercises that work different muscles of the large body parts and 2 to 3 different exercises that work different muscles of the small body parts. You can opt to do less of a variety of exercises, just be sure to add more sets.

Many believe that it is best to workout every other day. The downtime allows your muscles to rest. It is true that when muscles rest muscles repair and grow, however, on my plan you don't have to take days off between workouts, because you never work the same muscles more than once in a week. This gives you the flexibility to workout any 3 days of the week that fits best into your weekly schedule. I believe that devoting 3 out of 7 days a week to exercise is a fair number of days for those of you who do not want to live your lives in the gym. If after a while you find yourself wanting to workout more, by all means do so, but at the start I strongly suggest sticking to a maintainable number of days.

Now that you have an understanding of the weightlifting component of your workout routines, let's jump into some cardio!

Chapter 15

CARDIO

Cardio refers to any aerobic activities. This includes running and cycling, which can be done in or out of the gym. If you prefer group fitness programs, consider dance or other aerobics based classes. Contact sports such as football and hockey count toward cardio as well.

The benefit of cardio is that it raises the heart rate, speeds up metabolism and burns fat. I strongly suggest incorporating some form of cardio into your weekly workout routine.

Start by choosing which aerobic activities you'd like to include in your exercise routine. Next determine which days you'd like to do cardio. I suggest working cardio on the same days as your weightlifting exercises. If you are lifting weights at a gym it might be most convenient to run on a treadmill or cycle on a stationary bike to fulfill the cardio portions of your fitness routine. It's up to you.

In the beginning, limit your cardio to 3 days a week. If you find that in time you'd like to increase your aerobics, that is fine, however, I recommend 3 days, because it is maintainable number of days. All too often people are overly eager at the start, but can't keep up the pace, burn out and give up altogether.

No matter which aerobic activities you choose, be sure to pick one that you can execute for a minimum of 20 minutes a day. The trick in the beginning is to build your endurance. I've found that when most of my clients first start out, 20 minutes is a doable amount of time to work cardio, the goal is to work up to approx. 45 min cardio, yet I would rather see you jog on incline for 20 min. than walk for 45 min. on flat incline. It's all about intensity and sustainability.

On your workout days, I suggest weightlifting before cardio. Expend the majority of your energy on weightlifting, because it will burn more calories over time than cardio. You will burn calories during both weightlifting and cardio exercises, however, while at rest more calories will be burnt after a weightlifting session than aerobic activities.

An exception to the weightlifting before cardio rule is on the day of the week that you are working out your legs. Especially in the beginning, most find the leg workout to be intense and have difficulty running or cycling for 20 minutes or more following weight training.

One last important point about cardio is to be sure to incorporate warm up and cool down periods. For example, when you first step onto a treadmill start at a low setting and slowly increase your speed until you reach a comfortable pace. Before finishing your run, gradually decrease the speed. Warming up and cooling down before aerobic exercises puts less strain on your heart and helps to avoid pulled muscles or more severe injuries.

Chapter 16

CALISTHENICS

The third component to an optimal exercise and fitness routine is calisthenics. Calisthenics is muscle resistance training that can (but doesn't necessarily have to) involve weights and bands. Examples of calisthenics are pushups, sit-ups, squats, leg lifts etc.

Calisthenics are exercises that burn calories, while strengthening and conditioning muscles. When performing basic calisthenics exercises, such as pushups, you use your own body weight as resistance. With other forms of calisthenics, weights or bands can be used to increase tension resulting in a more difficult, yet effective workout.

Many of these exercises are simple, cost effective and can be performed in or out of a gym. If you are unable to afford a gym membership and don't have access to free-weights, calisthenics exercises can be used as a substitute to weightlifting.

Stomach Exercises
I strongly recommend incorporating calisthenics exercises that target stomach muscles into your 3-day workout routine. The stomach is a large body part that consists of four quadrants. The four quadrants of the stomach are upper right, upper left, lower right and lower left. Certain calisthenics exercises work all four quadrants, while others isolate muscles in one or more quadrants

Calisthenics exercises that effectively work stomach muscles include sit-ups and crunches. I incorporate sit-ups and/or crunches into my weekly exercise routines.

I begin my workouts by stretching and then move onto calisthenics exercises that target the stomach. Once those are complete, I typically move on to weightlifting exercises and then finish with cardio.

I've been at this for a while now, so on a typical workout day I complete at least 4 sets of 25 crunches and/or sit-ups targeting all 4 quadrants of the stomach. For beginners, set a realistic goal to strive for such as 4 sets of 10 sit-ups. You might find this to be an easily attainable goal. If so, that's great. Feel free to increase the number of sit-ups in each set. If you can't complete this initial goal number, it's fine. You're doing great. It's better to do less rather than push your limits, which could lead to you hurting yourself. Do what you can do and eventually you will reach your goal!

While performing sit-ups and/or crunches, be sure to exhale as you sit up and inhale as you lye back. Breathing is key. It is also important to take short rests in between each set. I usually take this time to stretch and relax.

Exercise and fitness, combined with dieting, will help you reach your goals and ultimately change your lifestyle.

PART III

LIFESTYLE

Chapter 17

SPORTS & ACTIVITIES

By now you understand the fundamentals of *The Model Body Plan*. Sticking to a solid diet and exercise routine can be challenging, however, it can also be a fun and rewarding process that could change your life forever.

Have you ever dreamed of running a marathon? Do you desire to become agile and flexible enough to master yoga? Does your lack of stamina impede on your ability to practice soccer or other sports with you kids? Does your current weight hold you back from enjoying your favorite amusement park rides? Do you get winded when you walk up a flight of stairs?

You can reach your goals and live a more satisfying life if you put your mind to it. Start by making small changes in your daily activities. The next time you have the option of taking an elevator versus walking up a few flights of stairs, choose the stairs. Looking for something to do on a sunny Sunday morning? Jump on a bicycle and take a ride through your neighborhood. It is fun and counts toward cardio. Instead of watching reality TV every night, create your own reality and sign up for a martial arts class.

The goal is to create healthier habits. The first attempt at change will be the most difficult, however, incorporating new sports and activities into your lifestyle will eventually become second nature to you. Staying active will increase your levels of serotonin, which could boost energy, aid in digestion and combat depression.

Chapter 18

REST & LEISURE

As important as it is to stay active, it is equally important to find adequate time for rest and relaxation. Sleep will help repair and rejuvenate your body. Participating in hobbies that you enjoy will clear your mind and help relieve stress.

Is there a particular book that you've been longing to read? Find a quiet garden or spot on the beach and escape in the story. Hear about a new film that interests you? Set plans with friends and head to the cinema. Been meaning to try out a new recipe? Take an afternoon off and cook a healthy meal for you and your family.

Choose hobbies that inspire and interest you. Are you a collector? Make time to sort coins, browse garage sales and flea markets or pursue consignment shops for that one of a kind purse. Ever dream of writing a novel? Set a plan and put that plan into action. Devote a specific amount of time each week and make your dream come true. Certain hobbies could lead to new professions, which could be life changing for you.

As you work toward creating a new lifestyle for yourself, it is extremely important to get adequate sleep. Six to eight hours a night is a healthy amount of rest. Personally, I feel most rested when I sleep for nine hours a night, however, my schedule doesn't always allow for me to do so. When I can't find time for my desired amount of sleep I try to squeeze in catnaps throughout the week. As children, naps were part of our daily routines, however, for some reason most adults replace naps with caffeine or other substances that push us to stay awake throughout the day. I opt rather to take a quick nap. A nap recharges my batteries. When I wake up, I feel refreshed and energized ready to continue my day in a positive and productive manner.

Chapter 19

BAD HABITS

The key to a healthy lifestyle is forming good habits. Staying active, participating in sports and activities and creating time for adequate rest and leisure will keep you balanced and in high spirits. As you work hard crafting the new you, do your best to steer clear of bad habits.

Alcohol

Alcoholic beverages, such as beer, will lead to weight gain unless you substitute it for a meal or the carbohydrate portion of your meal. If you want a beer with your burger, eliminate the fries. Take it one step further and eat your burger in a lettuce wrap instead of a bun. Remember, it's all about meeting your daily caloric intake goal. If you can eliminate beer altogether, that's great, but if not, be willing to sacrifice another food or beverage that day.

Liquor has calories as well. Whiskey, vodka and tequila have approximately 60-70 calories per ounce. These forms of alcohol can lead to dehydration (especially if you are not consuming adequate amounts of water). Do your best to avoid hard liquor altogether. You will be free of headaches and hangovers and your liver will thank you.

Certain alcoholic beverages (in moderation) are said to have positive effects on the body. Red wine, for example, contains antioxidants that could be good for the heart. If you opt for a glass of red wine, be sure to incorporate it into your daily caloric intake goal.

If you are one who craves white wine, I suggest mixing it with seltzer water. It's a refreshingly tasty beverage with half the calories.

I don't promote alcohol, infact it's the opposite but if you are going to drink, make sure you consult with your health care professional and If you are under 21 years old, don't drink!

Caffeine

Like alcohol, caffeinated beverages such as coffee and soda will dehydrate you. If you need that early morning coffee to jump start your day, consider drinking a bottle of water (instead of a soda) with lunch. I personally try to avoid caffeine, because it makes me feel nervous and jittery. While caffeine can suppress the appetite, there are healthier ways to diet. My best advice is to drink caffeinated beverages in moderation.

Smoking

We are all well aware of the dangers of smoking cigarettes and tobacco. Simply put, don't smoke, but if you do be sure to drink extra water throughout the day. Smoking dehydrates your body, which could leave you feeling weak and lethargic. While it might appear that a cigarette break relieves stress or gives you a burst of energy, the feeling is short lived. Overtime, your body will begin to crave the stimulant and you will find yourself in a negative pattern that will be extremely hard to break.

If you are a long time smoker there are many options to help you quit. Nicotine gum and patches (when used properly) can be useful tools to help you wean off smoking. Be sure to consult your doctor to determine which is the best option for you.

Don't be afraid of gaining weight when you quitting smoking. *The Model Body Plan* gives you full control over your weight and appearance. Take it one day at a time and try harder each day. You can do it!

Tanning

I grew up in a beach community, but I am not an advocate of tanning. Overtime, long exposures to the sun can be harmful to your body, dry your skin and leave you with a leathery, weathered appearance. Harmful ultraviolet (UV) rays emitted from the sun and tanning beds could cause skin cancer. Avoid tanning and wear sunscreen (even on overcast days). I suggest using a sunscreen that protects against both UVA and UVB rays. Many sunscreens are enriched with vitamins. Find a brand that works for you.

As you begin to reshape the new you, do your best to avoid bad habits. Start forming positive habits that you can enjoy throughout your life.

Chapter 20

HOLIDAYS & SPECIAL EVENTS

Sticking to your newly formed lifestyle will be challenging, especially during holidays, weddings and special events. Cut yourself a little slack! So often people beat themselves up during the holidays and in doing so it leads to feelings of guilt and depression. Remember that *The Model Body Plan* leaves room for flexibility. Try to stick to your daily caloric intake goal, but if you go over it's okay. It's better to enjoy your holiday or special event and wake up the next day with a positive mindset ready to jump back on track, rather than beat yourself up over eating a delicious piece of grandma's apple pie. You can always make up for it later in the week with a vegetable juice fast or extra day of cardio. It will all balance itself out in the end.

PART IV

INSPIRATION

Chapter 21

MOTIVATION

Now that you have the knowledge and tools you need to reach your goal, it's up to you to make the choices that will benefit your new lifestyle. Whether your goal is to simply loose weight, achieve a healthier lifestyle or sculpt your body into an ideal figure, you have the power to do so.

Ask yourself, what motivates me to reach my goal? I use to cut pictures of celebrities out of magazines and create collages and motivational boards. It was a visual reminder that would inspire me to reach my goals. Maybe you own a favorite outfit that you haven't been able to fit in for years. Look at that outfit everyday and visualize yourself wearing it. Don't you look stunning! Perhaps you'll be attending an event in the near future, such as a friend's wedding or a high school reunion, and you want to look your best. Make this your motivation. Whatever it is that inspires you is the right choice to keeping you on track to reaching your goals.

Chapter 22

MAINTENANCE

In the beginning, you might find my plan to be challenging at times, however, once you commit to it you will see results. Before you know it, you will reach your goal weight and then transition into the maintenance stage.

Maintaining your new weight is easier than loosing weight, because now you have room to play. For example, I encourage you to eat 4 meals a day as you work toward reaching your goal weight, however, you will have the flexibility to eat 2-6 meals a day once you have reached the maintenance stage. If you choose to eat an extra carbohydrate or happen to exceed your daily caloric intake goal on a holiday, it will be much easier to balance your calories out by eating less the next day.

Once you've reached the maintenance stage you will be conditioned and have the will to maintain your weight. This also applies to other lifestyle changes as well. You will be less likely to skip yoga class or drink a six-pack of beer, because you've worked so hard to reach your goal. You will find all aspects of your life that you've worked so hard to improve now easier to maintain.

In the next chapter you will read testimonials from people who have found success by following *The Model Body Plan*. Through hard work and dedication, they have reached and maintained their goals. If they can do it, so can you. I wish you the best of luck!

Chapter 23

TESTIMONIALS

"Through cutting portion sizes in half and being more conscious of my daily caloric intake, I have lost 15 lbs. and kept the weight off. Shedding pounds and achieving my ideal physique has boosted my confidence and inspired me to make many other lifestyle changes. I am booking more acting roles and modeling jobs than ever before. I believe in Aesha and The Model Body Plan so much that I volunteered to edit this book."

-- Chris Northrop

"With her determination and smart diet plan, Aesha helped me lose close to 80 lbs. Her rules are simple to follow. I am a whole new person now and would recommend this plan to anyone who is serious about losing weight."

-- Thea Samuelson

"I was more than 30 lbs. overweight. Though I exercised regularly, I lacked the will power to stick to any type of diet. I was feeling down on myself until I came across Aesha Waks's Model Body Plan. I began utilizing her simple nutrition plan and noticed changes immediately. I've already lost 12 lbs. and am going strong. I feel great and am more confident than I've felt in a long time. Best part is that I didn't have to

sacrifice burgers and other foods I love to accomplish my weight loss goals."

-- Stephen Steinberg

"Aesha is the most motivational and knowledgeable personal trainer that I've ever met. She tailored a unique workout and diet plan that has enabled me to maintain my weight and tone my body without ever having to compromise my lifestyle. Highly recommended!"

-- Miri Ben-Ari

PART V

4-WEEK JOURNAL

DIET JOURNAL

WEEK 1: DAY 1

<u>MEAL #</u>	<u>TIME</u>	<u>FOOD / DRINK</u>	<u>CALORIES</u>

Day 1 – Total Calories = _____

DIET JOURNAL

WEEK 1: DAY 2

MEAL #	TIME	FOOD / DRINK	CALORIES

Day 2 – Total Calories = _____

DIET JOURNAL

WEEK 1: DAY 3

MEAL #	TIME	FOOD / DRINK	CALORIES

Day 3 – Total Calories = _____

DIET JOURNAL

WEEK 1: DAY 4

MEAL #	TIME	FOOD / DRINK	CALORIES

Day 4 – Total Calories = _____

DIET JOURNAL

WEEK 1: DAY 5

MEAL #	TIME	FOOD / DRINK	CALORIES

Day 5 – Total Calories = _____

DIET JOURNAL

WEEK 1: DAY 6

<u>MEAL #</u>	<u>TIME</u>	<u>FOOD / DRINK</u>	<u>CALORIES</u>

Day 6 – Total Calories = _____

DIET JOURNAL

WEEK 1: DAY 7

MEAL #	TIME	FOOD / DRINK	CALORIES

Day 7 – Total Calories = _____

EXERCISE & FITNESS JOURNAL

WEEK 1: DAY 1

TYPE OF EXERCISE	# OF SETS	# OF REPS

EXERCISE & FITNESS JOURNAL

WEEK 1: DAY 2

TYPE OF EXERCISE	# OF SETS	# OF REPS

EXERCISE & FITNESS JOURNAL

WEEK 1: DAY 3

TYPE OF EXERCISE	# OF SETS	# OF REPS

LIFESTYLE JOURNAL

WEEK 1

What lifestyle change have I made this week?

INSPIRATIONAL JOURNAL

WEEK 1

What motivated or inspired me to stick to the plan this week?

How many pounds did I lose this week?

DIET JOURNAL

WEEK 2: DAY 1

MEAL #	TIME	FOOD / DRINK	CALORIES

Day 1 – Total Calories = _____

DIET JOURNAL

WEEK 2: DAY 2

MEAL #	TIME	FOOD / DRINK	CALORIES

Day 2 – Total Calories = _____

DIET JOURNAL

WEEK 2: DAY 3

MEAL #	TIME	FOOD / DRINK	CALORIES

Day 3 – Total Calories = _____

DIET JOURNAL

WEEK 2: DAY 4

MEAL #   **TIME**   **FOOD / DRINK**   **CALORIES**

Day 4 – Total Calories = _____

DIET JOURNAL

WEEK 2: DAY 5

MEAL #	TIME	FOOD / DRINK	CALORIES

Day 5 – Total Calories = _____

DIET JOURNAL

WEEK 2: DAY 6

MEAL #	TIME	FOOD / DRINK	CALORIES

Day 6 – Total Calories = _____

DIET JOURNAL

WEEK 2: DAY 7

MEAL #	TIME	FOOD / DRINK	CALORIES

Day 7 – Total Calories = _____

EXERCISE & FITNESS JOURNAL

WEEK 2: DAY 1

TYPE OF EXERCISE   **# OF SETS**   **# OF REPS**

EXERCISE & FITNESS JOURNAL

WEEK 2: DAY 2

TYPE OF EXERCISE   **# OF SETS**   **# OF REPS**

EXERCISE & FITNESS JOURNAL

WEEK 2: DAY 3

TYPE OF EXERCISE	# OF SETS	# OF REPS

LIFESTYLE JOURNAL

WEEK 2

What lifestyle change have I made this week?

INSPIRATIONAL JOURNAL

WEEK 2

What motivated or inspired me to stick to the plan this week?

How many pounds did I lose this week?

DIET JOURNAL

WEEK 3: DAY 1

MEAL #	TIME	FOOD / DRINK	CALORIES

Day 1 – Total Calories = _____

DIET JOURNAL

WEEK 3: DAY 2

MEAL #	TIME	FOOD / DRINK	CALORIES

Day 2 – Total Calories = _____

DIET JOURNAL

WEEK 3: DAY 3

MEAL #   TIME   FOOD / DRINK   CALORIES

Day 3 – Total Calories = _____

DIET JOURNAL

WEEK 3: DAY 4

MEAL #	TIME	FOOD / DRINK	CALORIES

Day 4 – Total Calories = _____

DIET JOURNAL

WEEK 3: DAY 5

MEAL #	TIME	FOOD / DRINK	CALORIES

Day 5 – Total Calories = _____

DIET JOURNAL

WEEK 3: DAY 6

MEAL #	TIME	FOOD / DRINK	CALORIES

Day 6 – Total Calories = _____

DIET JOURNAL

WEEK 3: DAY 7

MEAL #	TIME	FOOD / DRINK	CALORIES

Day 7 – Total Calories = _____

EXERCISE & FITNESS JOURNAL

WEEK 3: DAY 1

TYPE OF EXERCISE	# OF SETS	# OF REPS

EXERCISE & FITNESS JOURNAL

WEEK 3: DAY 2

TYPE OF EXERCISE   **# OF SETS**   **# OF REPS**

EXERCISE & FITNESS JOURNAL

WEEK 3: DAY 3

TYPE OF EXERCISE	# OF SETS	# OF REPS

LIFESTYLE JOURNAL

WEEK 3

What lifestyle change have I made this week?

INSPIRATIONAL JOURNAL

WEEK 3

What motivated or inspired me to stick to the plan this week?

How many pounds did I lose this week?

DIET JOURNAL

WEEK 4: DAY 1

MEAL #	TIME	FOOD / DRINK	CALORIES

Day 1 – Total Calories = _____

DIET JOURNAL

WEEK 4: DAY 2

MEAL #	TIME	FOOD / DRINK	CALORIES

Day 2 – Total Calories = _____

DIET JOURNAL

WEEK 4: DAY 3

MEAL #	TIME	FOOD / DRINK	CALORIES

Day 3 – Total Calories = _____

DIET JOURNAL

WEEK 4: DAY 4

MEAL #	TIME	FOOD / DRINK	CALORIES

Day 4 – Total Calories = _____

DIET JOURNAL

WEEK 4: DAY 5

MEAL #	TIME	FOOD / DRINK	CALORIES

Day 5 – Total Calories = _____

DIET JOURNAL

WEEK 4: DAY 6

MEAL #	TIME	FOOD / DRINK	CALORIES

Day 6 – Total Calories = _____

DIET JOURNAL

WEEK 4: DAY 7

MEAL #	TIME	FOOD / DRINK	CALORIES

Day 7 – Total Calories = _____

EXERCISE & FITNESS JOURNAL

WEEK 4: DAY 1

TYPE OF EXERCISE	# OF SETS	# OF REPS

EXERCISE & FITNESS JOURNAL

WEEK 4: DAY 2

TYPE OF EXERCISE	# OF SETS	# OF REPS

EXERCISE & FITNESS JOURNAL

WEEK 4: DAY 3

TYPE OF EXERCISE   **# OF SETS**   **# OF REPS**

LIFESTYLE JOURNAL

WEEK 4

What lifestyle change have I made this week?

INSPIRATIONAL JOURNAL

WEEK 4

What motivated or inspired me to stick to the plan this week?

How many pounds did I lose this week?

CONGRATULATIONS! You have successfully completed one month of *The Model Body Plan*. You're doing great! Take this time to reward yourself. I encourage you to keep up the good work. You will reach your goal weight before you know it!

Printed in the United States
By Bookmasters